Coconut Flour Recipes for Optimal Health and Quick Weight Loss

Gluten Free Recipes for Celiac Disease, Gluten Sensitivities, and Paleo Free Diets

Emma Rose

Table of Contents

Introduction

I want to thank you and congratulate you for purchasing this book.

This book contains proven steps and strategies on how to integrate coconut flour into your diet for a healthier food lifestyle.

In this book, you will learn about the benefits of using coconut flour and how it can help you lose weight and become healthier without limiting the food you're eating. I have also included several guilt-free coconut flour recipes that you and your loved ones will surely enjoy.

Thanks again for purchasing this book, I hope you enjoy it! Please take some time to stop by and LIKE our Facebook page:

https://www.facebook.com/joypublishing

With gratitude,

Emma Rose

Chapter 1: Why Use Coconut Flour?

Nowadays, people are getting more conscious about their food lifestyle and how it affects their overall well-being. Most of the foods that are available today are processed or refined however there are some good alternatives that can be used without taking away much from flavor.

Among the healthy alternatives for refined grains is the coconut flour. Coconut flour is one of the best alternatives to replace the usual refined wheat flour. Since coconut flour is very versatile, it can be used to replace refined grains from almost all kinds of baked goods and meals.

There are five major advantages in using coconut flour:

1. Coconut flour is gluten free. For people who have allergies or are sensitive to gluten, coconut flour is definitely a gift from heaven. By using coconut flour, people allergic to gluten will be able to enjoy baked treats.

2. Coconut flour improves cell regeneration. This type of flour has high non-gluten protein content that helps improve the growth of cells and rejuvenation.

3. Coconut flour is high in fiber. For people who want to lose or maintain their weight, coconut flour is a good alternative ingredient to make your own breads and cakes without feeling guilty about it. Foods made with coconut flour makes a person feel fuller faster and longer.

4. Coconut flour has high manganese content which means this ingredient will enable you to absorb more nutrients from foods faster. Also, manganese is proven to promote healthy blood sugar levels and thyroid health.

5. Coconut flour contains lauric acid. This healthy saturated fat is important to a person's immune health and it promotes healthy skin.

Though coconut flour can be used as a substitute ingredient to almost all recipes calling for wheat flour, it also takes some tweaking with the other ingredients for it to work well with baking and cooking. For example, coconut flour is drier than wheat flour therefore it requires more water when used in baking. The following are recipes that you can use to start your journey to a healthier you.

Chapter 2: Coconut Flour Bread Recipes

Zucchini Bread

Ingredients:

- ½ cup of coconut flour
- ¾ tsp of baking soda
- ½ tsp of salt
- 1 tbsp of cinnamon
- ½ tsp of nutmeg
- 4 pcs of pasture-raised eggs
- 3 tbsp of raw honey OR grade B maple syrup
- 1 cup of zucchini, shred it finely
- 1 pc of ripe banana, mashed
- 1 tbsp of coconut oil
- ½ cup of walnuts

Procedure:

1. Turn on the oven and set it to 350F.

2. Prepare a loaf pan and grease it with coconut oil. You can also line the pan with parchment paper, if available. Set the pan aside.

3. Prepare a piece of cheesecloth or a nut milk bag and place the finely shredded zucchini inside. Squeeze as hard as you can to remove the excess moisture from the zucchini.

4. In a large mixing bowl, combine the egg, honey or maple syrup, and banana. Mix together until the ingredients are well-incorporated.

5. Add in the coconut flour, baking soda, salt, cinnamon, and nutmeg into the mixing bowl and mix well. Then, add in the shredded zucchini and stir until the mixture becomes smooth.

6. Add in the walnuts and stir.

7. Pour the batter into the loaf pan and place it inside the oven. Bake for 45 to 50 minutes or until the bread has completely set.

Coco Doughnuts

Ingredients:

- ½ cup of coconut flour

- ¼ tsp of sea salt

- ¼ tsp of baking soda

- 6 pcs of eggs

- ½ cup of honey

- 1 tbsp of vanilla

- ½ cup of unsalted butter OR coconut oil, already melted

- 5 tbsp of honey

- Coconut flakes for toppings

Procedure:

1. Turn on the oven and set it to 350F.

2. In a mixing bowl, combine the coconut flour, sea salt, and baking soda. Stir the dry ingredients together until well-mixed.

3. Add in the eggs, honey, vanilla, and butter into the mixing bowl. Use a whisk or a hand mixer set on low to blend all of the ingredients together.

4. Prepare about 8 donut pan circles and fill each pan with the batter about 2/3 of the way.

5. Place the donut pan circles into the oven and bake for 20 minutes.

6. While baking, warm 5 tablespoons of honey and place it in a saucer. Then, toast the coconut flakes.

7. Dip each piece of donut in the honey and sprinkle it with the toasted coconut flakes.

Coco Bread

Ingredients:

- ¾ cup of coconut flour

- 1 tsp of baking soda

- A pinch of sea salt

- 4 pcs of whole eggs

- 3 pcs of eggs, white and yolk separated

- 5 tbsp of organic butter

- 3 tbsp of coconut milk

- 1 tbsp of raw honey

- Organic virgin coconut oil

Procedure:

1. Prepare a loaf pan and lightly grease it using the coconut oil. Then, line the loaf pan with baking paper with a coating of coconut oil just to make sure that the loaf does not stick to the pan.

2. Turn on the oven and set it to 350F.

3. Take the egg whites from three eggs and whisk it until it become stiff. You can use a hand mixer if you like. Set it aside.

4. Take the egg yolks and pour it in a food processor. Add in the four whole eggs, organic butter, coconut milk, and raw honey. Blend the ingredients until thoroughly combined.

5. Add in the coconut flour, baking soda, and salt gradually into the food processor while blending. Continue to process the ingredients until the mixture becomes thick in consistency.

6. Prepare a large mixing bowl and pour in the mixture from the food processor. Take the egg whites and fold it in the mixture.

7. Once the mixture and egg whites are thoroughly combined, pour in the batter into the loaf pan. Place the pan inside the oven and bake for 40 minutes.

8. Reduce the heat to 300F and cover the loaf pan. Cook for another 5 to 10 minutes.

9. Once cooked, remove the loaf pan from the oven and place it on a cooling rack to cool completely before slicing and serving.

Chocolate Muffin

Ingredients:

- ½ cup of coconut flour

- 1 tsp of baking soda

- A dash of salt

- ¼ cup of coconut sugar

- 2 tbsp of cocoa powder

- 1 tsp of vanilla extract

- ¼ cup of coconut oil

- 2/3 cup of coconut milk

- 4 pcs of pastured eggs

- 1 tsp of apple cider vinegar

Procedure:

1. Turn on the oven and set it to 350F.

2. Melt the coconut oil and place it in a bowl or a food processor. Add in the coconut flour, baking soda, salt, coconut sugar, cocoa powder, vanilla extract, coconut milk, eggs, and apple cider vinegar. Stir or blend the ingredients together until it forms a smooth batter.

3. Prepare a muffin tin and line it with paper or silicone liners.

4. Pour the batter about ¾ of the way of each muffin liner as the muffin will rise once it is cooked.

5. Place the muffin tin inside the oven and bake for 20 to 30 minutes.

Cheese Biscuits

Ingredients:

- 1/3 cup of coconut flour
- ¼ cup of butter, melted
- 4 pcs of eggs
- ¼ tsp of salt
- ¼ tsp of cream of tartar
- 1/8 tsp of baking soda
- ½ cup of shredded cheddar cheese
- ¼ cup of shredded parmesan cheese

Procedure:

1. Turn on the oven and set it to 400F.

2. In a mixing bowl, combine the coconut flour, salt, cream of tartar, and baking soda. Stir and make a well in the center of the dry ingredients.

3. Add in the eggs and melted butter in the center of the dry ingredients and mix. Whisk the ingredients together until it forms a smooth batter.

4. Add in the cheeses and stir to properly combine.

5. Prepare a baking sheet and spray it with cooking spray. Drop spoonfuls of batter into the sheet at even intervals.

6. Place the baking sheet inside the oven and bake for 8 to 10 minutes. Once cooked, let it cool on a wire rack then remove the biscuits from the baking sheet.

Gingerbread Doughnuts

Ingredients:

- 4 pcs of large eggs

- ¼ cup of melted coconut oil

- 1/3 cup of coconut palm sugar

- ¼ cup of full fat coconut milk

- 2 tbsp of blackstrap molasses (unsulphured)

- 1 tsp of raw apple cider vinegar

- 1 ½ tsp of pure vanilla extract

- 1 ¾ tsp of ground cinnamon

- 1 ¼ tsp of ground ginger

- 1 tsp of ground cloves

- ¾ tsp of allspice

- ½ tsp of baking soda

- ¼ tsp of freshly ground nutmeg

- ¼ tsp of sea salt

- 1/8 tsp of cayenne pepper

- ½ cup of coconut flour, sifted

- ½ cup of organic powdered sugar

- 2 tbsp of full fat canned coconut milk

- ¼ tsp of pure vanilla extract

- A pinch of sea salt

Procedure:

1. In a mixing bowl, combine the eggs, melted coconut oil, and palm sugar. Use a hand mixer to beat the ingredients together.

2. In a small bowl, combine the coconut milk, apple cider vinegar, molasses, and vanilla extract. Stir the ingredients together until properly combined. Pour the mixture into the large mixing bowl and beat until the ingredients are well mixed.

3. In a separate small bowl, combine the ground ginger, ground cloves, ground cinnamon, allspice, nutmeg, baking soda, cayenne pepper, and sea salt. Stir the ingredients together. Add in the spice mixture into the mixing bowl and stir until all the ingredients are just combined.

4. Add in the sifted coconut flour into the mixing bowl and use the hand mixer to incorporate all the ingredients. Blend until it forms a smooth batter.

5. Turn on the oven and set it to 350F.

6. Pour the batter into a doughnut pan and place it inside the oven. Bake for 18 to 20 minutes then place it immediately on a cooling rack.

7. While waiting for the doughnuts to cool, prepare a large mixing bowl and combine the organic powdered sugar, coconut milk, vanilla, and salt. Whisk the ingredients together until no lumps are present.

8. Use a spoon to drizzle the glaze over the doughnuts.

Lemon Bread with Lemon Glaze

Ingredients:

- 6 pcs of eggs

- ¼ cup of coconut oil, melted

- Zest of 2 pcs of lemons

- Juice from 2 lemons combined with coconut milk to make 1 cup

- 1/3 cup of honey

- 2/3 cup of coconut flour

- 1 tsp of baking soda

- ¼ tsp of salt

- 2 tbsp of coconut oil

- 2 tbsp of honey

- 2 tbsp of coconut milk

- Zest and juice of 1 lemon

- ½ tsp of vanilla extract

Procedure:

1. Turn on the oven and set it to 350F.

2. In a large mixing bowl, add in the eggs, ¼ cup of coconut oil, zest from 2 pieces of lemons, 1 cup of the lemon juice and coconut milk mixture, 1/3 up of honey, coconut flour, baking soda, and salt. Whisk the ingredients together until it forms a smooth batter.

3. Prepare a loaf pan and grease it with coconut oil. Pour the batter into the pan and place it inside the oven. Bake for 32 to 45 minutes then remove from the oven and set it aside to cool completely.

4. In a small bowl, combine the 2 tablespoons of coconut oil, 2 tablespoons of honey, 2 tbsp of coconut milk, zest and juice of 1 lemon, and vanilla extract. Whisk together until well-incorporated then pour the glaze on top of the loaf.

5. Place the loaf inside the refrigerator for about 30 minutes to help the glaze set before serving.

Chapter 3: Coconut Flour Breakfast Recipes

Coconut Porridge

Ingredients:

- ½ cup of full-fat canned coconut milk

- ¼ cup of water

- 3 tbsp of coconut flour

- 2 tbsp of finely shredded coconut

- ½ of a banana, mashed

- Frozen berries or chopped nuts, will be used for toppings

Procedure:

1. Prepare a small saucepan and add in the coconut milk, water, coconut flour, and the finely shredded coconut. Stir the mixture and let it boil.

2. Place a lid and reduce the heat. Let it simmer for 2 to 3 minutes stirring occasionally.

3. Remove the saucepan from the heat and add in the mashed banana. Whisk to combine and stir.

4. Replace the saucepan into the stove and cook for another 2 minutes. Continue stirring until it thickens.

Coconut Bake

Ingredients:

- 6 tbsp of coconut flour

- 10 pcs of eggs

- 2 tsp of vanilla extract

- 4 pcs of ripe bananas, mashed

- ¼ tsp of salt

Procedure:

1. In a mixing bowl, add in the coconut flour, eggs, vanilla extract, mashed bananas, and salt. Mix the ingredients thoroughly and let it sit for 10 minutes.

2. Prepare a muffin tin by lining it with muffin liners. Then, pour the batter into the tin.

3. Place the muffin tin inside the oven and bake for 20 to 25 minutes at 350F. You can also bake this in your microwave for 3 minutes on high settings. Just remember to use ramekins instead of muffin tins.

Bacon Pancakes

Ingredients:

- 16 pcs of cooked bacon strips

- ¼ cup of mashed ripe banana

- 4 pcs of large eggs

- 6 tbsp of full fat canned coconut milk

- 1 tsp of apple cider vinegar

- 1 tsp of vanilla extract

- 3 tbsp of organic coconut flour

- 1 tsp of cinnamon

- ½ tsp of baking soda

- A pinch of salt

- Coconut oil

- 2 tbsp of maple syrup

Procedure:

1. Place the bacon on a wire rack and bake it in the oven for 10 to 20 minutes at 400F.

2. In a medium mixing bowl, combine the mashed banana, eggs, apple cider vinegar, coconut milk, and vanilla. Whisk the ingredients together until properly combined.

3. In a separate mixing bowl, combine the organic coconut flour, baking soda, cinnamon, and salt. Give it a stir until the ingredients are incorporated.

4. Pour in the banana mixture into the coconut flour mixture and whisk together until the batter has no lumps.

5. Prepare a skillet and heat the coconut oil. Once the oil is hot, add in three tablespoons of batter into the pan. Make a rectangular shaped pancake about the size of your bacon. Flip the pancake once bubbles form on top.

6. Repeat the process until all the batter is cooked then assemble the pancakes. Place strips of bacon on top of a pancake then drizzle with a bit of maple syrup. Put another pancake on top and enjoy.

Strawberry Flapjacks

Ingredients:

- 1 pc of egg

- 1 tbsp of almond flour

- 1 tsp of coconut flour

- Coconut oil

- ¼ tsp of baking soda

- ½ tsp of cream of tartar

- Stevia

- Organic strawberries

Procedure:

1. Prepare a skillet and heat the coconut oil.

2. In a small bowl, whisk the egg and adding in a splash of water. Once combined, add in the almond flour and coconut flour and whisk again.

3. Add in the baking soda, stevia, and cream of tartar. Mix the ingredients together until it forms a smooth batter. You can taste the batter to gauge the amount of stevia needed.

4. Slice the strawberries into thin slices.

5. Pour the batter into the pan to make one mini-pancake. Once the pancake is slightly firm, place strawberry slices on top. Flip the pancake to cook the other side.

Oats and Flax Crisps

Ingredients:

- 2/3 cup of rolled oats

- 1/3 cup of flax seeds

- ½ cup of shredded coconut

- ¼ cup of coconut oil, melted

- 1/3 cup of unsweetened coconut milk

- 3 tbsp of maple syrup

- 2 tbsp of coconut flour

- 1 tbsp of coconut sugar

- 1 tbsp of chia seeds

- 3 tsp of ground ginger

- 1 tsp of cinnamon

- 1 tsp of pure vanilla extract

- ¼ tsp of salt

Procedure:

1. Turn on the oven and set it to 350F. Prepare two baking sheets and line it with silicone mats or parchment paper.

2. In a large mixing bowl, combine the rolled oats, flax seeds, shredded coconut, coconut flour, coconut sugar, chia seeds, ground ginger, cinnamon, and salt. Stir the ingredients together until evenly combined.

3. In a separate bowl, combine the coconut oil, coconut milk, maple syrup, and vanilla extract. Stir the ingredients until well-mixed. Then, pour the mixture over the dry ingredients. Stir the ingredients together until properly incorporated.

4. Drop a spoonful of the mixture into the baking sheets and flatten it with the back of the spoon to make thin biscuit-like crisps.

5. Place the baking sheets in the oven and bake for 18 to 25 minutes. Once cooked, remove the baking sheets from the oven and set it aside to cool completely.

Chapter 4: Coconut Flour Cake Recipes

Apple and Cinnamon Cake

Ingredients:

- 6 pcs of free-range eggs

- 1 cup of coconut oil OR organic butter, already melted

- ¼ cup of raw honey

- 1 pc of apple, grated

- Zest of 1 pc of lemon

- ½ cup of coconut flour

- 1 cup of desiccated coconut

- 2 tsp of cinnamon

- 1 tsp of baking soda

- A pinch of sea salt

- 1 pc of apple, slice it into very thin wedges

- Juice of ½ of a lemon

- Extra coconut flour for dusting

Procedure:

1. Turn on the oven and set it to 150C.

2. Prepare a cake tin and spray it with cooking oil. You can also line it with parchment paper if you prefer.

3. In a food processor, add in the eggs, coconut oil, honey, grated apple, lemon zest, coconut flour, desiccated coconut, cinnamon, baking soda, and sea salt. Blend all of the ingredients together until properly combined.

4. Spoon the batter into the cake tin and spread it evenly.

5. Arrange the wedges of apples on top of the batter. Decorate it however you like. Then, squeeze the lemon juice on the apples.

6. Place the cake tin inside the oven and bake for 45 minutes.

7. Once cooked, let it cool complete before transferring it into a serving plate. Dust with the extra coconut flour before serving.

Coffee Cake

Ingredients:

- 1 cup of coconut flour

- ½ tsp of Celtic sea salt

- 1 tsp of ground cinnamon

- 8 pcs of large organic eggs

- 1 tsp of baking soda

- ½ cup of strained plain coconut milk yogurt

- 5 tbsp of coconut oil

- ½ cup of honey

- 1 tbsp of vanilla extract

- 1 ½ cups of nuts

- 2 tsp of cinnamon

- 4 tbsp of honey

- 4 tbsp of cold coconut oil, cut it into tablespoons

Procedure:

1. Turn on the oven and set it to 325F. Place the rack in the middle part of the oven.

2. In a food processor, combine the coconut flour, sea salt, 1 teaspoon of ground cinnamon, eggs, baking soda, coconut milk yogurt, 5 tablespoons of coconut oil, ½ cup of honey, and vanilla extract. Blend the ingredients until the mixture becomes smooth.

3. Prepare an 8" x 8" baking dish and pour in the batter inside.

4. Wash and dry the food processor bowl. Add in your choice of nuts, 2 teaspoons of cinnamon, 4 tablespoons of honey, and 4 tablespoons of coconut oil. Process until the nuts are coarsely chopped and all of the ingredients bind together.

5. Spoon the topping on the batter and spread it across the surface of the batter.

6. Place the baking dish in the oven and bake for 40 to 45 minutes. Once cooked, place it on a wire rack and let it cool for about 20 minutes before cutting and serving.

Chocolate Cake

Ingredients:

- ¾ cup of coconut flour, sifted
- ¼ cup of cacao powder
- 1 tsp of Celtic sea salt
- 1 tsp of baking soda
- 10 pcs of eggs
- 1 cup of coconut oil
- 1 ½ cups of coconut sugar
- 1 tbsp of vanilla extract
- ¼ tsp of orange zest
- 1 cup of dark chocolate
- ½ cup of grapeseed oil
- 2 tbsp of agave nectar
- 1 tbsp of vanilla extract
- A pinch of Celtic sea salt

Procedure:

1. In a small mixing bowl, combine the coconut flour, cacao powder, Celtic sea salt, and baking soda. Mix the ingredients together.

2. In a large mixing bowl, combine the eggs, coconut oil, coconut sugar, vanilla extract, and orange zest. Use a hand mixer to mix the ingredients until properly incorporated.

3. Gradually add in the dry ingredients mixture into the large bowl while blending with the hand mixer.

4. Prepare two 9" round cake pans. Lightly grease it with oil and dust using the coconut flour. Pour the batter inside the cake pans and place it inside the oven.

5. Set the oven to 325F and bake for 35 to 40 minutes.

6. Once cooked, remove from the oven and place it on a cooling rack to cool completely.

7. Prepare a small saucepan and add in the dark chocolate and grapeseed oil. Combine the two ingredients over low heat.

8. Add in the agave nectar, vanilla extract, and salt into the saucepan. Stir until the ingredients are well-incorporated.

9. Remove from the heat and place it inside the freezer for about 15 minutes.

10. Once cool, remove the frosting from the freezer and use the hand mixer to whip the frosting until it becomes thick and fluffy.

11. Place the frosting in between the two layers of cakes. Place one cake on top of the other and use the remaining frosting to cover the top of the cake.

Double Chocolate Beet Root Brownies

Ingredients:

- 4 pcs of large pastured eggs

- 1/3 cup of coconut oil, melted

- 1 tsp of vanilla extract

- ¾ cup of maple syrup

- 1 ½ cups of beet puree

- 2 tbsp of coconut cream

- ½ cup of coconut flour

- ½ cup of raw cocoa powder

- ½ tsp of unrefined salt

- ½ tsp of baking soda

- ½ cup of chocolate chips

Procedure:

1. Turn on the oven and set it to 350F.

2. In a large mixing bowl, combine the eggs, coconut oil, vanilla extract, maple syrup, beet puree, and coconut

cream. Use a hand mixer to thoroughly mix the ingredients.

3. In another bowl, combine the coconut flour, cocoa powder, salt, baking soda, and chocolate chips. Stir to mix the ingredients together.

4. Gradually add in the dry ingredients into the large mixing bowl containing the wet ingredients. Use the hand mixer to properly combine the ingredients.

5. Prepare an 8" x 8" baking pan and grease it lightly with coconut oil. Then, pour the batter into the pan.

6. Place the baking pan inside the oven and bake for 35 to 40 minutes.

Pumpkin Bars

Ingredients:

- 1 ½ cups of pumpkin puree

- ¾ cup of coconut flour

- ¾ cup of maple syrup

- 1 ½ tsp of ground cinnamon

- ¾ tsp of ground ginger

- ¼ tsp of ground cloves

- ¾ tsp of baking soda

- ¼ tsp of salt

- 2 pcs of large eggs

- Coconut oil

Procedure:

1. Turn on the oven and set it to 350F.

2. Prepare a 9" x 9" baking dish and lightly grease it using the coconut oil.

3. In a large mixing bowl, combine the pumpkin puree, coconut flour, maple syrup, ground cinnamon, ground

cloves, ground ginger, baking soda, salt, and eggs. Stir the ingredients together until well-incorporated.

4. Pour the batter into the baking dish and smooth the top. Place the baking dish inside the oven and bake for 40 to 45 minutes. Once cooked, let it cool completely before cutting and serving.

Chocolate Chip Banana Cookies

Ingredients:

- 1 pc of ripe banana

- 1 pc of large egg

- 2 tbsp of extra virgin coconut oil

- 3 tbsp of coconut flour, sifted

- 1 tbsp of vanilla extract

- ½ tsp of cream of tartar

- 1/8 tsp of baking soda

- 1/8 tsp of sea salt

- ¼ cup of chocolate chips

Procedure:

1. Turn on the oven and set it to 325F.

2. Prepare a baking pan and line it with parchment paper.

3. In a large mixing bowl, combine the banana and egg. Use a hand mixer to mix the ingredients together. Slowly add in the coconut oil while mixing.

4. Add in the coconut flour, vanilla extract, cream of tartar, baking soda, and sea salt. Blend the ingredients until it forms a smooth batter.

5. Add in the chocolate chips into the batter and stir.

6. Use a spoon to drop about 1 inch balls of batter on the baking pan then flatten the batter to form a cookie shape. Leave enough space between each cookie.

7. Place the baking pan inside the oven and bake for 40 minutes.

Classic Vanilla Cake

Ingredients:

- 4 pcs of large eggs, whites and yolks separated

- 1 tsp of cream of tartar

- ¼ cup of extra virgin coconut oil

- 3 tbsp of raw honey

- ¼ cup of coconut flour, sifted

- 2 tsp of vanilla extract

- ¼ tsp of baking soda

- 1/8 tsp of salt

Procedure:

1. Turn on the oven and set it to 350F.

2. Prepare an 8" x 1.5" round cake pan and line it with parchment paper.

3. In a large mixing bowl, combine the cream of tartar with the egg whites. Use a whisk or a hand mixer to whip the ingredients together to form stiff peaks.

4. In a separate mixing bowl, combine the honey and coconut oil. Use a hand mixer to mix the two

ingredients to form a cream. Add in the egg yolks, and mix again.

5. Gradually add in the coconut flour, vanilla extract, baking soda, and salt into the mixture. Use the hand mixer to combine the ingredients until it forms a smooth batter.

6. Pour the batter into the bowl with the whipped egg whites and fold until properly incorporated. Pour the mixture into the cake pan.

7. Place the cake pan in the oven and bake for 20 minutes.

Lady Finger Cookies

Ingredients:

- 4 pcs of pastured eggs, separate the white from the yolk

- ¼ cup of maple syrup

- ¼ tsp of baking soda

- ½ tsp of vanilla extract

- 1/3 cup of coconut flour, sifted

- 1 tsp of freshly ground coffee

Procedure:

1. Turn on the oven and set it to 400F.

2. Place the egg whites in a mixing bowl and beat it until stiff peaks form using a hand mixer.

3. In a large mixing bowl, add in the egg yolks, vanilla extract, baking soda, and maple syrup. Whisk the ingredients together until properly combined. Add in the sifted coconut flour and continue to mix the ingredients until it forms a smooth batter.

4. Fold the egg whites into the mixture then add in the ground coffee.

5. Prepare a baking sheet and line it with parchment paper. Pour the batter into a pipe bag and attach a

round pipe tube at the end. Make about 3-in long cookies on the baking sheet.

6. Place the baking sheet inside the oven and bake for 13 minutes. Once down, set it aside to cool completely before serving.

Custard Cake

Ingredients:

- 4 pcs of eggs

- 2 cups of milk

- ½ cup of coconut flour

- ½ cup of raw honey

- 1 tsp of pure vanilla extract

- 2 tsp of baking powder

- ¼ cup of butter, melted

- 1 ½ cups of unsweetened coconut flakes

- ½ cup of chocolate chips

Procedure:

1. Turn on the oven and set it to 350F.

2. In a large bowl, add in the eggs, coconut flour, milk, honey, vanilla extract, baking powder, and butter. Whisk the ingredients together until it forms a smooth batter. You can use a hand mixer if you prefer.

3. Add in the chocolate chips and coconut flakes. Stir until all ingredients are properly combined.

4. Prepare an 8" cake pan and pour the batter inside. Place the pan inside the oven and bake for 45 to 50 minutes.

5. Once cooked, let it rest and cool completely before splicing and serving.

Conclusion

Thank you again for purchasing this book.

I hope this book was able to help you to discover the benefits of using coconut flour.

The next step is to enjoy the recipes you have learned to make healthier foods for yourself and your loved ones.

Losing weight and changing your lifestyle isn't easy. We all need motivation to keep our goal in mind.

Finally, please remember to check out our Facebook page in order to find other resources and upcoming promotions:

https://www.facebook.com/joypublishing

With sincere thanks,

Emma Rose

Preview of "The Almond Flour Recipes for Optimal Health and Quick Weight Loss: Gluten Free Recipes for Celiac Disease, Gluten Sensitivities, and Paleo Free Diets"

Chapter 1: Almond Flour

Almond is native to the northern Indian subcontinent. The almond seed is more of a drupe than a nut. Like peaches, cherries and apricots, almond trees bears fruits with seeds inside which are commonly referred to as almond nut.

Almond flour is a popular substitute to wheat flour in baking and cooking. This is made from whole almonds with the skins removed. This is often preferred by health conscious individuals because it is gluten-free, high in fiber and low in carbohydrates. It is also an excellent source of protein. Almond flour is also rich in vitamins and minerals including magnesium, potassium and vitamin E.

Benefits of using almond flour:

Nutrients

Almond flour contains Vitamin E which can help prevent cell damage and heart disease. It also contains calcium which strengthens the bone and helps your circulatory system carry hormones throughout your body. Almond flour is also rich in potassium which can regulate your blood pressure.

Easy to Prepare

You can purchase almond flour in your local grocery or make it yourself. Just submerge the almonds in boiling water for a minute. Place in a strainer and remove the skin. Allow to dry then place in a coffee grinder or food processor. Process until it becomes very fine.

Complementary Foods

Serving dishes and pasties with almond flour can supplement the protein that you get from meat. It also balances your diet if it is served with fruits and vegetables. Almond flour can also compliment gluten free and low carbohydrate diets.

Reduces Heart Disease Risk

Almond contains high amounts of monounsaturated fats. This is the type of fat found in olive oil which is associated with good heart health. The antioxidants in the almond flour can also help keep the arteries healthy.

Chapter 2: Bread and Pancakes

Paleo Pumpkin Bread

Ingredients:

- 1 cup blanched almond

- ½ tsp baking soda

- 1 tsp nutmeg

- ½ cup roasted pumpkin

- ¼ tsp stevia

- ¼ tsp Celtic sea salt

- 1 tbsp ground cinnamon

- ½ tsp cloves

- 2 tbsp honey

- 3 large eggs

Procedure:

1. Combine the spices such as cinnamon, cloves, nutmeg, and cloves along with the almond flour and salt in a food processor.

2. Blend few times then add the stevia, pumpkin, eggs and honey.

3. Transfer the batter into a loaf pan.

4. Bake for 45 minutes at 350 degrees.

5. Allow to cool for an hour before slicing.

6. Serve alone or with your favorite spread.

Check out the rest of "Almond Flour Recipes for Optimal Health and Quick Weight Loss: Gluten Free Recipes for Celiac Disease, Gluten Sensitivities, and Paleo Free Diets" on Amazon.

Or go to: http://amzn.to/1qx2LaT

Check Out My Other Books

Below you'll find some of my other books also available on Amazon and Kindle. Search for these titles on the Amazon website to find them.

Paleo Free Diet Guide for Beginners: Over 50 Paleo Free Recipes for Optimal Health & Fast Weight Loss

Paleo Desserts: Satisfy Your Sweet Tooth With Over 100 Quick & Easy Paleo Dessert Recipes & Paleo Baking Recipes

Raw Food Diet Guide: Lose Weight Quickly, Achieve Optimal Health & Feel Energized with the Raw Food Diet & Raw Food Recipes

Clean Eating Guide: Lose Weight Quickly, Achieve Optimal Health & Feel Energized with Clean Eating For Busy Families & Clean Eating Recipes

Alkaline Diet Guide: Lose Weight Quickly, Achieve Optimal Health & Feel Energized with the Alkaline Diet & Alkaline Recipes

Coconut Flour Recipes for Optimal Health & Quick Weight Loss: Gluten Free Recipes for Celiac Disease, Gluten Sensitivities & Paleo Free Diets

Almond Flour Recipes for Optimal Health & Quick Weight Loss: Gluten Free Recipes for Celiac Disease, Gluten Sensitivities & Paleo Free Diets

Wheat Free Diet for Beginners: Lose Weight Quickly, Achieve Optimal Health & Feel Energized with Gluten Free Recipes for Celiac Disease, Gluten Sensitivities & Paleo Free Diets

Detox Diet Guide: Lose Weight Quickly, Achieve Optimal Health & Feel Energized Through the 10 Day Detox

Sugar Detox Guide for Beginners: Lose Weight Quickly, Achieve Optimal Health, Feel Energized & Eliminate Sugar Cravings Naturally

Ketogenic Diet Guide for Beginners: How to Achieve Rapid Weight Loss, Optimal Health & Unstoppable Energy with Ketogenic Diet Recipes

Anti Inflammatory Diet for Beginners: Lose Weight Fast, Optimize Health, Slow Aging, Fight Inflammation, Conquer Pain & Increase Energy with the Anti Inflammation Diet Recipes

One Last Thing...

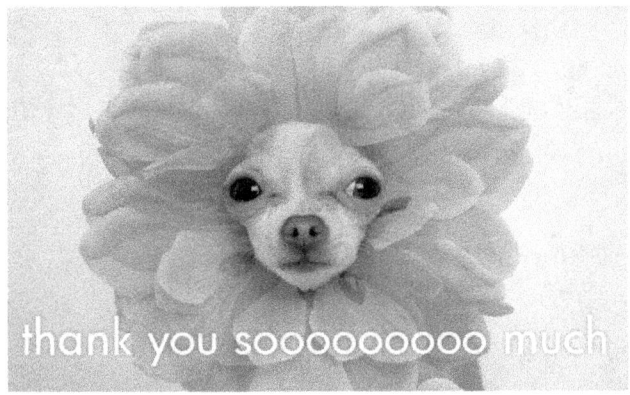

thank you sooooooooo much

If you believe that this book is worth sharing, would you please take the time to let others know how it affected your life? If it turns out to make a difference in the lives of others, they will be forever grateful to you, as will I.